# BRIAN DIET RECEIPT FOR SENIORS

**SUBTITLE:** A Brain-Boosting Culinary Guide for Seniors

## BY: BRIAN BRAIN

Copyright [c] 2023
BRIAN BRAIN

All rights reserved. no part of this publication may be copied, or transmitted in any form or by any means, including photocopying, recording, or other electronic or mechanical methods, without the consent of the copyright holder, except in the case of agreed quotations in critical reviews and certain other uses permitted by copyright law.

# TABLE OF CONTENTS:

# INTRODUCTION:

My grandmother found comfort in the delicate hands who cared for her in the quiet corridors of the care home, where soft whispers and loving smiles replaced the rush and bustle of the outside world. It was a place where stories echoed in every room, where memories whispered through the corridors, and where the human spirit was evident. But, in the middle of dementia's struggles, my family and I discovered an unexpected source of hope and healing - a recipe not only for the body, but also for the soul.

Several years ago, as my grandmother began her dementia journey, our family was faced with the difficult duty of assuring her well-being and quality of life. Witnessing the gradual loss of her once-vibrant personality was sad, and we were determined to find a way to bring her peace, enjoyment, and a sense of purpose. In the midst of our hunt for answers, we came across a simple yet significant remedy - a healthy meal that not only filled her body but also regenerated her spirit.

The narrative began with a dedicated caregiver in the nursing home, someone who saw beyond the illness and remembered the person my grandmother used to be. This caring lady, equipped with a thorough understanding of nutrition and a true affection for the patients she cared for, set out on a quest to develop meals adapted to their specific requirements. One day, she introduced us to a cuisine that would become a cornerstone of my grandmother's journey to wellness - a dish that went beyond ordinary food, becoming a beacon of light in the face of hardship.

This recipe, carefully made with healthful ingredients and filled with love, transformed dinner into a treasured tradition. Its perfume flooded the air, luring my grandmother to the dining table with a renewed sense of expectation. With each bite, we saw a spark in her eyes, a glimpse of recognition, and a flicker of the joy that dementia had tried to take away. It was more than simply food; it was a lifeline, linking her to the world she was slowly leaving behind.

As we implemented this specific recipe into her regular routine over the next few months, a surprising shift occurred. The nourishing elements not only improved her physical condition but also seemed to reawaken dormant sections of her memory. Conversations grew more coherent, smiles more frequent, and moments of clarity became more valuable. The simple act of sharing a meal created a bridge, allowing us to connect with the essence of who she was outside the limits of her situation.

As our family witnessed the wonderful impact of this healthful and mindful approach to meal preparation, we recognized we had discovered something incredibly powerful. The event sparked a desire in us to learn more about the connection of diet and dementia care. We conducted research, consulted with specialists, and learnt about the tremendous impact of particular nutrients on brain health and cognitive function. With this information, we became champions for a holistic approach to dementia care, highlighting the importance of personalized, nourishing meals in the lives of those impacted by this difficult condition.

In the pages that follow, I encourage you to accompany me on a journey of knowledge, compassion, and transformation. We will investigate the science behind diet and dementia, share inspiring stories of resilience, and learn how to prepare healthy, tasty meals that nourish not only the body but also the soul. This is a monument to the wonderful power of food, love, and human connection - a recipe for wellness that transcends illness and reminds us of the extraordinary resilience of the human spirit.

# CHAPTER 1:

## DEMENTIA, TYPES, SYMTOMS, CAUSES AND PREVENTIVE MEASURES:

Dementia is a catch-all term for a verity of cognitive impairments that interfere with daily life and functioning. It is not a sickness in and of itself, but rather a syndrome marked by a decline in memory, reasoning, behavior, and capacity to execute daily tasks. Dementia affects millions of individuals globally, making it a major public health concern.

Alzheimer's disease is the most common type of dementia, accounting for approximately 60-80% of cases.

Other types of dementia include vascular dementia, which is caused by decreased blood supply to the brain, and Lewy body dementia, which is characterized by aberrant protein deposits in brain cells. Frontotemporal dementia affects the frontal and temporal lobes of the brain, causing personality and behavioral abnormalities. Each variety of dementia has its own set of symptoms and progression patterns, but they all have one thing in common: cognitive loss.

The symptoms of dementia differ based on the type and stage of the disease. Memory loss, disorientation, and difficulty finding the proper words or understanding discussions are common early warning symptoms. Individuals with dementia may face difficulties with problem solving, changes in attitude and behavior, and difficulty doing familiar tasks as the disease develops. Individuals in advanced phases may lose the ability to identify family members and struggle with basic self-care duties.

The specific origins of dementia are unknown, but research indicates that a mix of genetic, environmental, and lifestyle factors may play a role. Age is a major risk factor, with the likelihood of acquiring dementia increasing with age. Furthermore, some genetic variations and a family history of dementia can increase the risk. Chronic disorders like cardiovascular disease, diabetes, and high blood pressure all have a role in the development of vascular dementia. Injuries to the brain, illnesses, and exposure to environmental pollutants may all raise the risk.

While there is no treatment for dementia, there are preventive strategies and lifestyle choices that can help reduce the risk and postpone the start of symptoms. Regular physical activity has been found to boost brain health and lower the risk of dementia. A healthy, well-balanced diet high in antioxidants, omega-3 fatty acids, and vitamins promotes cognitive performance. Mental stimulation, such as puzzles, reading, or acquiring new skills, can help to keep the brain active and resilient. Managing cardiovascular risk factors, such as keeping a healthy weight, controlling blood pressure, and not smoking, can also help with overall brain health.

To summarize, dementia is a complex and difficult disorder that affects millions of people globally. Understanding the many forms, detecting the symptoms, and implementing preventive measures are critical steps in solving this worldwide health issue. Individuals may make informed choices to promote brain health and improve the quality of life for those affected by dementia and their families thanks to ongoing research and growing understanding.

# CHAPTER 2:

## MEALS TO EAT AND AVOID:

It's critical to focus on nutrient-dense foods that support brain health and overall well-being when creating a nutritious meal plan for dementia sufferers, while avoiding products that can accelerate cognitive decline.

**Foods to Consume:**

**Fatty fish**: such as salmon, trout, and sardines, are high in omega-3 fatty acids, which enhance brain function and may prevent cognitive decline.

**Colorful Vegetables:** Antioxidants and vitamins found in colorful vegetables such as broccoli, kale, and bell peppers protect the brain from oxidative stress.

**Berries:** Blueberries, strawberries, and blackberries are high in antioxidants, which help to preserve memory and cognitive functions.

Walnuts, almonds, flaxseeds, and chia seeds provide healthful fats, antioxidants, and vitamin E, which promote brain function.

Whole grains, such as brown rice, quinoa, and whole wheat, provide a continuous supply of energy to the brain.

**Lean Proteins:** Consume lean meats, poultry, eggs, and lentils to support muscular health and keep blood sugar levels steady.

Low-fat dairy or fortified plant-based substitutes provide calcium and vitamin D, which are essential for bone health and overall well-being.

**Avoid these foods:**

**Saturated and trans fats:** Limit your consumption of fried foods, processed snacks, and fatty cuts of meat, as these foods linked to heart disease and cognitive decline.

**Excess Sugar:** Excess sugar consumption has been linked to inflammation and may impair cognitive performance; restrict sweets, sugary beverages, and processed desserts.

Foods heavy in preservatives, sodium, and artificial additives should be avoided since they might have a negative impact on overall health.

Excess salt can cause high blood pressure, increasing the risk of vascular problems; avoid processed foods and salty snacks.

Excessive alcohol use can exacerbate cognitive impairment; moderation is necessary, or it may be advisable to avoid alcohol entirely.

Individuals can maintain maximum health, cognitive function, and overall well-being in the face of dementia by emphasizing a diet rich in brain-boosting nutrients and avoiding dangerous drugs.

# CHAPTER 3:

## BENEFIT FOR MAINTAIN A HEALTHY DEMENTIA MEAL:

A dementia-specific diet has various advantages for seniors, improving their general well-being and quality of life. Here are the main benefits:

**Cognitive Assistance:**

Improved Brain Function: Nutrient-dense meals such as fatty fish, berries, and leafy greens include critical vitamins and antioxidants that promote brain health and cognitive function. **2. Emotional Stability: Omega-3 fatty acids present in fish assist sustain brain cell structure and function, potentially preventing cognitive decline.

**Blood Sugar Balance:** Whole grains, lean proteins, and foods with a low glycemic index help to manage blood sugar levels, minimizing severe spikes and falls. Stable blood sugar levels help to maintain mood stability and prevent irritation and disorientation.

**Physical Fitness:**

Heart Health: A dementia diet rich in fruits, vegetables, and lean meats has been shown to benefit cardiovascular health. This is critical because what is healthy for the heart is also excellent for the brain, lowering the risk of strokes and cognitive deficits caused by vascular disease.

Weight Control: A well-balanced diet aids in the maintenance of a healthy weight, lowering the risk of obesity-related illnesses such as diabetes and hypertension, both of which are known risk factors for dementia.

## Digestive Wellness:

Fiber-Rich Foods: Whole grains, fruits, and vegetables are high in fiber, which promotes regular bowel movements and prevents constipation, a major problem among seniors.

## Power and stamina:

Muscle Health: Adequate protein intake from sources such as lean meats, eggs, and legumes promotes muscle health, ensuring seniors' strength and mobility as they age.

Consistent Energy: Whole grain complex carbs give a steady energy supply, minimizing energy slumps and supporting everyday activities.

## Improved Hydration:

Incorporating Hydrating Foods: Foods high in water content, such as cucumbers, watermelon, and soups, aid in hydration, which is essential for overall health and mental clarity.

## Better Digestive and Absorption:

Avocados and almonds, for example, are high in healthy fats, which aid in the absorption of fat-soluble vitamins, ensuring seniors get the most nutritional value from their meals.

## Better Quality of Life:

Sharing meals and helping to prepare dementia-friendly foods can be a social activity that improves emotional well-being and provides a sense of purpose.

Reduced Stress for caretakers: A well-nourished senior may demonstrate enhanced behavior and cognitive capacities, decreasing stress for both the individual and their caretakers.

Incorporating a dementia-specific diet suited to the needs of seniors is a comprehensive approach that not only addresses cognitive health but also supports their physical, emotional, and social well-being, thereby improving their overall quality of life.

# CHAPTER 4:

## COMPLICATIONS THAT MAY ARISE IF THE PROPER MEAL IS NOT FOLLOWED:

If individuals with dementia do not maintain a correct and nutritious diet, various issues might occur, worsening the difficulty connected with the condition:

**Malnutrition:** Patients suffering from dementia may forget to eat or have trouble eating independently. Malnutrition can result, producing weakness, exhaustion, and a compromised immune system, leaving them more prone to infections and other ailments.

**Dehydration:** Individuals with dementia may struggle to stay hydrated due to forgetfulness or cognitive problems. Dehydration increases the risk of urinary tract infections, renal issues, and falls due to dizziness and weakness.

**Weight Loss:** A lack of appetite, trouble swallowing, or forgetting to eat can lead to severe weight loss, which can contribute to muscle weakness and a weakened immune system. Severe weight loss can also impair the body's capacity to regulate temperature, making it more susceptible to illness.

**Cognitive Decline:** In dementia patients, a shortage of critical nutrients, particularly those that maintain brain health, can hasten cognitive decline. Proper diet is critical for sustaining brain function and delaying illness progression.

**Increased Behavioral and Psychological Symptoms:** Decreased nutrition can cause increased irritability, agitation, and hostility, all of which are prominent behavioral symptoms in dementia patients. A healthy diet can help control these symptoms as well as improve general happiness and well-being.

Bone Health Concerns: Inadequate calcium and vitamin D intake can result in weakening bones, increasing the risk of fractures and falls, which can be especially harmful for seniors with dementia.

**Impaired Immune Function:** Malnutrition impairs the immune system, making dementia patients more susceptible to infections such as respiratory illnesses and urinary tract infections, which can result in hospitalization and additional health concerns.

**Gastrointestinal Issues:** Poor nutrition can induce gastrointestinal problems such as constipation, which can be uncomfortable and increase behavioral symptoms in dementia patients.

Proper nutrition suited to the specific needs of people with dementia is critical for avoiding these consequences. Caregivers and healthcare professionals play an important role in ensuring that dementia patients eat nutritious, well-balanced meals that address not only their physical health but also their cognitive and emotional well-being.

# CHAPTER 5:

## HEALTHY MEAL PLANNING FOR DEMENTIA, BENEFIT AND PROPER PLANNING:

Healthy meal planning for dementia is an important part of managing the condition, as it provides various benefits that help to the general well-being and quality of life of those living with dementia. Here's how a well-planned meal plan may make a big difference:

## Customized Nutritional Needs:

Balanced Diet: A varied diet rich in antioxidants, omega-3 fatty acids, vitamins, and minerals promotes brain health, prevents cognitive decline, and preserves physical health.

Foods High in Protein: Adequate protein consumption is essential for muscle strength and repair. Incorporating lean meats, poultry, fish, eggs, and plant-based proteins into your diet promotes general health and mobility.

## Cognitive Assistance:

Brain-Boosting Foods: Consuming antioxidant-rich foods like berries and leafy greens, as well as omega-3 fatty acids from fatty fish, improves cognitive performance and memory recall.

## Water intake:

Hydrating Foods: Including hydrating foods like high-water-content fruits and clear soups in the diet helps prevent dehydration, which is frequent in dementia patients and can lead to a variety of issues.

## Digestive Wellness:

Fiber-Rich Diet: Whole grains, fruits, and vegetables are high in fiber, which promotes regular bowel movements and prevents constipation, a major problem among seniors.

## Behavioral and Emotional Stability:

Low glycemic index foods, such as whole grains and legumes, assist maintain stable blood sugar levels, minimizing mood swings, irritability, and behavioral disorders.

## Weight Control:

**Portion Control:** Maintaining a healthy weight, lowering the risk of obesity-related diseases, and ensuring individuals have enough energy without consuming too many calories are all benefits of proper portion control.

**Emotional and social connection:**
Meal Sharing: Mealtime may be a social and joyful event. Sharing meals with family or friends strengthens emotional bonds and creates a sense of belonging, which improves general well-being.
Support for caregivers:

Simplified Meal Preparation: Meal plans developed for simplicity of preparation benefit caregivers by ensuring that they can deliver nutritious and well-balanced meals without undue stress.
Caregivers can receive help on designing suitable food plans, boosting their capacity to properly serve their loved ones.
In conclusion, dementia management requires a carefully designed and nutritionally balanced diet. It not only

covers physical health but also cognitive function, emotional well-being, and general quality of life for both the person with dementia and their caregivers. Proper meal planning adapted to the specific needs of individuals with dementia can considerably enhance their general health and ability to manage with the conditions problems.

Certainly! Here are seven recipes for dementia-friendly breakfasts, each with its components, preparation method, quantity, nutritional value, and estimated cooking time:

## 1. Almond-Blueberry Oatmeal

Ingredients:

a half-cup rolled oats

1 cup water or milk (vegan or dairy)

1 cup blueberries, fresh

1 tablespoon almonds, chopped

1 teaspoon (optional) honey or maple syrup

1 tsp cinnamon

## Value for money:

Fiber, antioxidants, and healthy fats are abundant. Essential vitamins and minerals are provided.

**Preparation:**
Combine the oats and water or milk in a saucepan. Cook, stirring periodically, for 5 minutes, or until the oats are soft and creamy.

Cook for 2 minutes more, or until the blueberries burst and release their juices.

Remove from the heat and place in a mixing basin.

Top with chopped almonds, honey or maple syrup, and cinnamon, if desired. Serve immediately.
Cooking time: 7 minutes

# 2. Berry Yogurt Parfait

## Ingredients:
1 cup strained Greek yogurt
1/2 cup berry mixture (strawberries, blueberries, raspberries)
2 tbsp. granola
1 tbsp. honey
1 teaspoon chia seeds

## Value for money:
Protein, probiotics, antioxidants, and fiber are abundant. Essential vitamins and minerals are provided.

**Preparation:** Layer half of the Greek yogurt on the bottom of a glass or bowl.

On top of the yogurt, arrange a layer of mixed berries.

Half of the granola should be sprinkled on top of the berries.

Repeat with the rest of the yogurt, berries, and granola.

If used, drizzle with honey and top with chia seeds.

Serve immediately or store in the refrigerator for later.

Cooking Time: None


**Smoothie with Banana and Nuts**

**Ingredients:**
1 banana (ripe)
a half-cup Greek yogurt
1/4 cup chopped nuts

1 tablespoon maple syrup or honey
1/2 cup milk (dairy or soy)
1 tsp vanilla extract

## Value for money:

Potassium, protein, healthy fats, and vitamins and minerals are all present.

## Preparation:

Blend banana, Greek yogurt, chopped almonds, honey or maple syrup, milk, and vanilla extract in a blender until smooth.

Blend till creamy and smooth.
Pour into a glass and top with chopped nuts.

Immediately serve.

Cooking Time: None

# Scrambled Eggs with Vegetables

## Ingredients:
2 eggs
1/4 cup chopped (assorted colors) bell peppers
14 cup spinach, chopped
halved 1/4 cup cherry tomatoes
season with salt and pepper to taste
a tsp olive oil

## Value for money:
Protein, fiber, vitamins, and minerals are all abundant. Essential fatty acids are provided.

## Preparation:
Heat olive oil in a nonstick skillet over medium heat.

Sauté the diced bell peppers until slightly tender.

Sauté for another minute with the cherry tomatoes and spinach.

Whisk together eggs, salt, and pepper in a mixing bowl.

Combine the eggs and vegetables in a skillet.

Cook until the eggs are fully cooked and scrambled, stirring carefully.

Transfer to a platter after removing from the heat. Serve warm.
Time to cook: 5-7 minutes


## 5. Yogurt and Fruit Pancakes


### Ingredients:
1/2 cup pancake mix (whole grain)
1/2 cup water or milk (vegan or dairy)
a half-cup Greek yogurt

1/2 cup fresh fruits (strawberries, bananas, blueberries, etc.)
1 tablespoon maple syrup or honey

**Value for money:**
Fiber, protein, vitamins, and minerals are all included. Sugars are kept to a minimum.

**Preparation:**

per make the pancake batter, combine whole grain pancake mix and water or milk in a mixing bowl, according per package directions.

Over medium heat, heat a nonstick griddle or skillet.

To make a pancake, pour a tiny amount of batter onto the griddle.

Cook the pancake until bubbles appear on the surface, then turn and cook until golden brown on both sides.

To make more pancakes, repeat with the remaining batter.

Serve the pancakes topped with Greek yogurt and a variety of fresh fruits.

Drizzle with maple syrup or honey. Serve immediately.

Cooking time: 10-15 minutes (for numerous pancakes)

## 6. Fruit and Cottage Cheese Salad

**Ingredients:**
1/2 cup cottage cheese, low-fat

1/2 cup fresh fruit mix (e.g., pineapple pieces, melon, or grapes)
1 tbsp chopped nuts (almonds, pistachios)
1 tsp honey

**Value for money:**
Protein, calcium, antioxidants, and vital vitamins are all abundant.

**Preparation:** Combine cottage cheese and assorted fresh fruits in a bowl.
Top with chopped nuts.
Drizzle with honey to taste.
To blend, gently toss everything together.
Serve cold.

Cooking Time: None

## 7. Breakfast Wrap With Veggies

## Ingredients:

1 tortilla (whole grain)
2 fried eggs
1/4 cup chopped (assorted colors) bell peppers
1 cup diced tomatoes
14 cup spinach, chopped
season with salt and pepper to taste
1 tablespoon salsa

## Value for money:

Protein, fiber, vitamins, and minerals are all included. Saturated fats are little.

## Preparation:

Cook diced bell peppers, chopped tomatoes, and chopped spinach in a nonstick skillet until soft.

Season with salt and pepper if desired.

Scramble the eggs until fully done in the same skillet.

In the skillet, warm the whole grain tortilla for a few seconds on each side.

Spread the scrambled eggs evenly across the tortilla.
Top the eggs with the sautéed veggies.
Add a tablespoon of salsa if desired.
Fold the tortilla sides over the filling to form a wrap.

Serve immediately.

Time to cook: 5-7 minutes

These dishes are intended to be healthful, simple to prepare, and appealing to dementia patients. Caregivers can change the textures and flavors based on the individual's tastes and nutritional needs. Always seek the advice of a healthcare practitioner or a nutritionist to ensure that the recipes meet any dietary demands or restrictions.

# CHAPTER 7:

## 7 DAYS HEALTHY LUNCH MEAL PLAN:

Certainly! Here are seven dementia-friendly lunch recipes, each with its components, preparation method, quantities, nutritional value, and cooking time estimate:

**Stir-Fry with Salmon and Vegetables**

**Ingredients:**
1 salmon fillet (about 4 oz)
1 cup sliced mixed vegetables (bell peppers, broccoli, carrots)
1 tablespoon soy sauce (low sodium)
1 tablespoon extra virgin olive oil
1 garlic clove, minced. Brown rice, cooked (optional, for serving)
**Value for Money:**

Omega-3 fatty acids, protein, and antioxidants are abundant. It contains important vitamins and minerals.

**Preparation:**
Make bite-sized pieces of the salmon fillet.

In a skillet over medium heat, heat the olive oil. Sauté the minced garlic until fragrant.

Cook until the salmon becomes opaque and flakes easily with a fork.

Stir in the mixed vegetables until they are cooked but still somewhat crunchy. To incorporate, drizzle with low-sodium soy sauce and stir.

If desired, serve over cooked brown rice.

Time to cook: approximately 10 minutes

**Salad with Quinoa and Chickpeas**

**Ingredients:**
1 cooked cup quinoa
1/2 cup washed and drained canned chickpeas
1/4 cup cucumber, diced
1/4 cup halved cherry tomatoes
2 tbsp fresh parsley, chopped
1 tablespoon extra virgin olive oil
Half a lemon juice. Season with salt and pepper to taste.
**Value for Money:**
Protein, fiber, vitamins, and minerals are abundant. Saturated fats are scarce.

**Preparation:**

Combine cooked quinoa, chickpeas, sliced cucumber, cherry tomatoes, and chopped parsley in a mixing dish.

Drizzle with olive oil and lemon juice, to taste.

Toss with salt and pepper until well combined.

Refrigerate for 30 minutes before serving to let flavors to develop.

Cooking Time: About 15 minutes (for cooking quinoa)

**Stir-Fry Chicken with Vegetables**

**Ingredients:**

1 thinly sliced boneless, skinless chicken breast
1 cup sliced mixed vegetables (bell peppers, snap peas, carrots)
2 tbsp teriyaki sauce (low sodium)
1 tablespoon extra virgin olive oil (Optional) cooked brown rice or whole grain noodles (for serving)

## Value for Money:
Protein, fiber, vitamins, and minerals are abundant. Saturated fats are scarce.

## Preparation:
In a skillet over medium heat, heat the olive oil. Cook until the chicken is no longer pink in the center.

Stir in the mixed vegetables until they are cooked but still somewhat crunchy.

Pour the teriyaki sauce with low sodium over the chicken and vegetables. Stir thoroughly to coat evenly.

If desired, serve over cooked brown rice or whole grain noodles.

Time to cook: approximately 15 minutes

**Wrap with turkey and avocado**

**Ingredients:** 1 whole wheat tortilla
3 ounces thinly sliced cooked turkey breast
1/4 sliced avocado
1 tablespoon mixed greens (spinach, lettuce)
1 tbsp Greek yogurt or light mayonnaise
Season with salt and pepper to taste.

**Value for Money:**

Protein, healthy fats, fiber, and vitamins are all included.

**Preparation:**
Place the whole grain tortilla on a flat surface.

Spread the tortilla equally with Greek yogurt or low-fat mayonnaise. On one side of the tortilla, layer turkey slices, avocado slices, and mixed greens.

Season to taste with salt and pepper.

To make a wrap, roll the tortilla tightly.

To make eating easier, cut the wrap in half diagonally.

Cooking Time: None required

# Stir-Fry with Vegetables and Tofu

## Ingredients:

1/2 firm tofu block, diced
1 cup sliced mixed vegetables (bell peppers, snow peas, mushrooms)
2 tbsp stir-fry sauce with low sodium
1 tbsp sesame seed oil
1/2 teaspoon ginger, minced
Brown rice, cooked (optional, for serving)

## Value for Money:
Protein, fiber, antioxidants, and vital vitamins are abundant.

## Preparation:
To remove extra moisture, press the tofu between paper towels. Cut the potatoes into cubes.

In a skillet over medium heat, heat the sesame oil. Sauté the minced ginger until aromatic. Cook until the tofu cubes are golden brown on all sides.

Stir in the mixed vegetables until they are cooked but still somewhat crunchy.

Serve the tofu and vegetables with the low-sodium stir-fry sauce. Stir thoroughly to coat evenly.

If desired, serve over cooked brown rice.

Time to cook: approximately 15 minutes

## Sandwich with Egg Salad

**Ingredients:**
2 peeled and sliced hard-boiled eggs
2 tbsp plain Greek yogurt
1/4 cup celery, chopped
1 tablespoon fresh chives, chopped
Season with salt and pepper to taste.
Slices of whole grain bread

**Value for Money:**
Protein, healthy fats, and important vitamins and minerals are all present.

**Preparation:**
Combine chopped hard-boiled eggs, Greek yogurt, diced celery, and chopped chives in a mixing dish.

Season to taste with salt and pepper. To construct a sandwich, spread the egg salad mixture onto slices of whole grain bread.

For added freshness, add lettuce or spinach leaves.

To finish the sandwich, add another slice of bread.

Time to cook: about 10 minutes (for boiling eggs)

**Salad with Chickpeas from the Mediterranean**

**Ingredients:**

1 can (15 oz) washed and drained chickpeas
1 cup diced cucumber
1/2 cup halved cherry tomatoes
1/4 cup finely chopped red onion
1/4 cup pitted and sliced Kalamata olives
2 tbsp fresh parsley, chopped

2 tablespoons crumbled feta cheese
2 tbsp of olive oil
Half a lemon juice
Season with salt and pepper to taste.

## Value for Money:

Protein, fiber, antioxidants, and healthy fats are abundant. It contains important vitamins and minerals.

## Preparation:

Combine chickpeas, diced cucumber, cherry tomatoes, red onion, Kalamata olives, and chopped parsley in a large mixing basin.

Drizzle with olive oil and lemon juice, to taste.

Toss with salt and pepper until well combined.

Before serving, top with crumbled feta cheese.

Refrigerate for 30 minutes before serving to let flavors to develop.

Cooking Time: None required

These dishes are intended to be healthful, simple to prepare, and appealing to people suffering with dementia. Caregivers can change the textures and flavors based on individual preferences and dietary needs. To verify that the recipes meet specific dietary demands and restrictions, always consult with a healthcare practitioner or a nutritionist.

**1. Baked Chicken with Lemon Herbs
Ingredients:**

a single (6 ounce) chicken breast

One-third cup olive oil

one-tsp of new lemon juice

One tspn dried herbs (oregano, thyme, or rosemary)

To taste, add salt and pepper.

**Value for Nutrition:**

Rich in vital minerals, lean protein, and vitamin C.

**Get ready:** Set oven temperature to 375°F, or 190°C. Put the chicken breast in the ovenproof dish.

Combine the olive oil, lemon juice, dried herbs, salt, and pepper in a small bowl.

Ensure that the chicken is evenly coated by pouring the liquid over it.

Bake until the chicken is cooked through, 25 to 30 minutes.

Warm up and serve.

Cooking Time: About 25 to 30 minutes

## 2. Vegetable Stuffed Bell Peppers with Quinoa

Additives:

Two bell peppers, seeded and cut in half One-half cup cooked quinoa Diced 1/2 cup of mixed vegetables (spinach, tomatoes, and zucchini).

1/4 cup grated feta cheese

One-third cup olive oil

Half a tspn dried herbs of Italy

To taste, add salt and pepper.

**Value for Nutrition:**

abundant in vitamins, minerals, fiber, and antioxidants.

**Get ready:**

Set oven temperature to 375°F, or 190°C.

Put the cooked quinoa, mixed veggies, feta cheese, dried herbs, olive oil, and salt and pepper in a bowl. Place the quinoa mixture inside the bell pepper halves.

Stuff the peppers and arrange them in a baking dish.

The peppers should be baked for 20 to 25 minutes, or until soft.

Warm food is served.

Cooking Time: 20 to 25 minutes on average


## 3. Foil packets with salmon and asparagus

Additives:

One 6-ounce salmon fillet

Cup of blanched asparagus spears

One-third cup olive oil

1 tablespoon finely sliced fresh dill one minced clove of garlic

To taste, add salt and pepper. Lemon wedges as a garnish

**Value for Nutrition:**

Rich in protein, antioxidants, and omega-3 fatty acids.

**Get ready:**

Warm the oven up to 400°F, or 200°C.

The salmon fillet should be placed on foil.

Combine asparagus, minced garlic, olive oil, dill, salt, and pepper in a bowl.

Place the asparagus on top of the salmon.

Make sure the packet is sealed by folding the foil.

Bake until the salmon is cooked through, 15 to 20 minutes.

Serve after garnishing with slices of lemon.

Preparation Time: 15 to 20 minutes

## 4. Chickpea Curry without Meat

Additives:

One fifteen-ounce can of rinsed and drained chickpeas

One cup of mixed vegetables (peas, tomatoes, and bell peppers)

one-half cup coconut milk

Curry powder, one tablespoon

One-third cup olive oil

one minced clove of garlic

To taste, add salt and pepper.

To garnish, use fresh cilantro.

## Value for Nutrition:

Packed with fiber, vital minerals, and plant-based protein.

**Get ready:**

Olive oil should be heated in a skillet over medium heat. Once the garlic is minced, sauté it until aromatic.

Stir for two to three minutes after adding the chickpeas and mixed veggies.

Over the veggies and chickpeas, sprinkle curry powder. Well combine.

Once added, simmer for ten to fifteen minutes. Add pepper and salt according to taste.

Before serving, add some fresh cilantro as a garnish.

Serve with quinoa or rice, if preferred.

Preparation Time: 15 to 20 minutes

## 5. Turkey Hash with Sweet Potatoes

Additives:

Turkey ground, half a pound

Peel and dice one medium sweet potato.

chop half a cup of onions

half a cup of chopped bell peppers

One-third cup olive oil A half-teaspoon of paprika smoked

To taste, add salt and pepper.

As a garnish, fresh parsley

Value for Nutrition:

gives nutritious carbohydrates, lean protein, and vital vitamins.

**Get ready:**

Olive oil should be heated in a skillet over medium heat. Add chopped onion and cook it until it turns transparent.

Break the ground turkey into little bits with a spoon as you cook it until it turns brown.

Add the bell peppers and diced sweet potato. Simmer until the sweet potato is soft.

Over the mixture, scatter the smoked paprika. Make a good stir.

Add pepper and salt according to taste.

Before serving, sprinkle some fresh parsley on top.

Warm up and serve.

Cooking Period: 15 minutes or so

## 6. Omelette with mushrooms and spinach

Additives:

Two oeufs

half a cup of sliced mushrooms cut half a cup of fresh spinach

1/4 cup grated feta cheese

One-third cup olive oil

To taste, add salt and pepper.

**Value for Nutrition:**

Rich in iron, vitamins, and protein.

**Get ready:**

Add salt and pepper to a bowl and whisk the eggs.

In a nonstick skillet set over medium heat, warm the olive oil.

Add the sliced mushrooms and cook them until their moisture evaporates.

After adding, boil the spinach until it wilts.

Over the spinach and mushrooms, pour the whisked eggs.

Top with feta cheese that has been crumbled.

Once the edges become firm, fold the omelette in half.

Warm up and serve.

Cooking Period: About 8 to 10 minutes

## 7. Soup with Lentils and Veggies

Additives:

1 cup well-rinsed dry lentils

1 cup diced mixed veggies (carrots, celery, and tomatoes)

chop half a cup of onions

one minced clove of garlic

Four cups of broth made with vegetables One-third cup olive oil

One tsp. of dried thyme

To taste, add salt and pepper.

**Value for Nutrition:**

Rich in fiber, vegan protein, and a range of vitamins.

**Get ready:**

Olive oil should be heated over medium heat in a big pot. Saute the minced garlic and chopped onion until they become tender.

Add the mixed vegetables and simmer for two to three minutes.

Add the washed lentils and pour in the vegetable broth.

Season with pepper, salt, and dry thyme. After bringing the soup to a boil, lower the heat, and simmer it for 25 to 30 minutes, or until the lentils become soft.

Warm up and serve.

Preparation Time: About.

# CHAPTER 9:

## CONCLUSSION:

In summary, this dementia disease cookbook acts as a kind manual that provides not only recipes but also a vital source of assistance for people with dementia and the people who care for them. We hope that these well considered dishes will not only nourish but also comfort you, making every meal an opportunity to improve your physical and emotional health.

A thorough study of the particular dietary requirements of those suffering from dementia has been the driving force behind the development of these recipes. These meals emphasize entire, nutrient-dense foods and specially prepared cooking techniques to support mental and physical well-being and improve overall quality of life.

Beneath the delectable recipes contained in these pages is a deeply inspirational story of perseverance and hope. Every dish is an ode to the healing power of food for both body and mind, showing that the act of cooking and sharing a healthy meal can bring comfort and strength to anybody facing difficult circumstances.

We offer a unique incentive to the reader: accept these recipes as instruments to promote happiness, connection, and wellbeing rather than merely following recipe instructions.

Accept the kitchen as a creative and therapeutic environment where all ingredients have the power to improve lives and produce special moments. Accept the chance to take care of yourself and your loved ones, knowing that every wholesome meal you take today is a step toward a better, happier tomorrow.

I hope these dishes warm your heart and nurture your body, serving as a reminder that despite life's obstacles, there is a world of flavor, coziness, and love just waiting to be experienced. Accept the transforming force of these meals, and allow them to serve as a lighthouse pointing you in the direction of a future full of life, relationships, and the endless pleasures of communal, healthful eating.

www.ingramcontent.com/pod-product compliance
Lightning Source LLC
Chambersburg PA
CBHW050847260726
48660CB00006B/2488